Badra Bahri
Ines Sdiri

Failure of non-invasive ventilation in covid patients 19

Badra Bahri
Ines Sdiri

Failure of non-invasive ventilation in covid patients 19

Clinical aspects and predictive factors

ScienciaScripts

Imprint

Cover image: www.ingimage.com

This book is a translation from the original published under ISBN 978-620-6-72294-6.

Publisher:
Sciencia Scripts
is a trademark of
Dodo Books Indian Ocean Ltd. and OmniScriptum S.R.L publishing group

120 High Road, East Finchley, London, N2 9ED, United Kingdom
Str. Armeneasca 28/1, office 1, Chisinau MD-2012, Republic of Moldova, Europe
Printed at: see last page
ISBN: 978-620-8-31125-4

CONTENTS

INTRODUCTION

COVID-19 is an infectious disease caused by a new coronavirus, SARS-CoV-2 (severe acute respiratory syndrome coronavirus 2), an enveloped single-stranded RNA virus responsible for respiratory infections. mainly low-lying with variable manifestations (1).

It has rapidly become a global health emergency and from a first declared on 1[er] December 2019 in China (2), the World Health Organisation has qualified it as a pandemic in March 2020 with over 100 countries affected. (3)

This new and emerging disease was characterised by an epidemiological evolution in successive waves. This was explained by the mutagenic power of the virus, creating different epidemiological profiles from one country to another, with different clinical presentations.

Symptoms can range from a mild form with a simple cough and flu-like symptoms, to severe forms causing acute respiratory failure (ARF) that can progress to acute respiratory distress syndrome. These severe forms require intensive care, with frequent recourse to mechanical ventilation (non-invasive or invasive). (4)

According to an international cohort conducted between 30 January 2020 and 5 January 2022, including 700,000 patients from 70 countries, 16% of patients required admission to intensive care and 61.3% required invasive ventilation (2). In these patients, in-hospital mortality was high (3).

Since the first case was identified in Tunisia on 02 March 2020, our country has seen a rapid rise in the number of cases, leading to saturation of emergency and intensive care services. Up to October 2022, there will be 1.15 million cases of COVID 19 in Tunisia, with more than 30,000 deaths (2).

This particular development of COVID 19 has led to the need (both internationally and nationally) for a dynamic and progressive approach to management that adapts to the different clinical pictures presented. Initially, in the absence of a well-defined consensus and the availability of different ventilation devices, ventilatory management differed from one team to another. Some teams recommended invasive mechanical ventilation (IMV) from the outset to limit the risk of aerosolisation and contamination. Others opted for non-invasive ventilation (NIV) as a first-line treatment, with recourse to invasive ventilation in the event of failure (4) .

Currently, for most teams, non-invasive ventilation remains the reference ventilatory technique, in particular the SV-AI-PEP mode (5). Its aim is to avoid the need for invasive mechanical ventilation, which is associated with a high mortality rate (3). In the absence of recommendations, the timing and criteria for intubation are generally left to the discretion of the clinician(6). As a result, the decision to intubate may sometimes be delayed, with the risk of worsening pulmonary lesions and patient prognosis. This can have a negative impact on the results of non-invasive or even invasive strategies, with high mortality in critically ill COVID-19 patients (7,8). While several studies have demonstrated the efficacy of non-invasive ventilation (11), others have attempted to define the factors that predict its failure (6).

A better understanding of the factors leading to NIV failure could enable intensive care units to establish dynamic management of this serious pathology, in order to guarantee optimal and appropriate care. The aim of our study was to describe the epidemiological, clinical, radiological and therapeutic characteristics, as well as the ventilatory strategy, of patients hospitalised with severe COVID19 pneumonia, and to identify factors predictive of NIV failure.

METHODS

1. Type and location of study

This is a descriptive, retrospective, mono-centric study conducted in the emergency and medical intensive care unit of the Habib Thameur Hospital in Tunis, over a period from 07/07/2020 to 31/12/2020.

2. Location the study

The study was carried out in the emergency and intensive care unit of the Habib Thameur Hospital in Tunis, which is a university hospital with several medical and surgical specialities but no pulmonology department.

The Emergency and Intensive Care Department is a multi-purpose unit. It has an emergency unit, a medical intensive care unit with a capacity of 8 beds, and an intensive care unit for patients admitted with a COVID 19 infection with a capacity of 13 beds.

This is the COVID 19 reference service at hospital level since the start of the COVID 19 pandemic in 2020.

3. Population studied

3.1 Inclusion criteria

➢ Patients with a COVID 19 infection in its critical form according to the INEAS definition (April 2021) and hospitalised for more than 48 hours.

➢ Over 18 years of age

➢ Use of non-invasive ventilatory support

3.2 Non inclusion criteria

- Patients admitted with non-critical COVID 19
- All patients with a length of stay of less than 48 hours.
- Use of invasive ventilation from the outset

3.3. Exclusion criteria

-Missing files.

4. judgement criteria

The primary outcome was failure of NIV and use of invasive mechanical ventilation.

The secondary endpoint was mortality.

5. Collection of data

For each patient included in the study, data were collected on a standardised form **(Appendix 1)**, based on medical records, monitoring sheets and hospitalisation reports (progress, investigations, computerised medical record).

The parameters collected were :

5.1. Data anamnestic

- Patient identification: surname, first name, gender and date of birth.
- Personal history: age, medical history.
- Functional signs prior to admission to the intensive care unit
- Pre-admission consultation

5.2. Clinical signs

- The temperature
- Physical examination
- Signs of respiratory distress

5.3. Paraclinical data

5.3.1. Biological data

- Arterial blood gas analysis (ABG)

- Blood count.
- D-Dimer and fibrinogen assays
- Renal function data,
- Inflammation data (CRP and procalcitonin levels)
- Results of bacteriological sampling.

5.3.2. Data from tomodensitometry

- The percentage of parenchymal involvement was estimated according to a 5-grade visual classification (9,10), as well as the presence or absence of associated pulmonary embolism.
- We also described the presence or absence of images suggestive of COVID involvement: ground glass, crazy-paving and condensation.
- Presence of signs of fibrosis and possible pathological lung.

5.4. Coverage

5.4.1 Support ventilation

Ventilatory management was based on several modes (11):

- Simple oxygen therapy
- Non-invasive ventilation (NIV) in SV-AI-PEP or CPAP mode, its parameters and duration.
- Optiflow-type high-flow nasal oxygen therapy (HFO), its parameters and duration.
- Invasive mechanical ventilation (IMV), its parameters and duration

5.4.2 Prone position

Prone decubitus (PD) is a simple technique recommended for the treatment of severe hypoxemia in ARDS, and consists of turning the patient into PD. There are four main stages in this manoeuvre:

- **Preparing the patient :**

- Take haemodynamic and respiratory vitals.
- Carrying out eye care and occlusion.
- Carry out mouth and nose care.
- Ensure that probes are securely attached and check that catheters are patent.
- Protect the chin and knees with a hydrocolloid dressing.

- **Turn the patient over** (with three or five carers depending on the patient's build):

- Place the patient on his or her side, using the sheet underneath.
- Remove the electrodes from the chest.
- Place a new sheet on the patient's bed.
- Turn the patient onto their stomach and centre them.

- **Resettle the patient:**

- Replace the electrodes on the patient's back.
- Protect pressure points with artificial skin such as Duoderma to prevent bedsores.
- Position the patient's head on its side and vary the position every 3 hours.
- Position the patient's arms: the arm opposite the intubation at eye level and the other at the side of the body.
- Position the patient's legs on a pillow (level with the shins).
- Position the probes and drains and check the patency of the vascular approaches.
- Check the permeability of airwaysairways and perform a if necessary.
- Recline the bed in the procline position to 20°.

• Take haemodynamic and respiratory vitals.

5.4.2. Support haemodynamics

Haemodynamic support was necessary in patients in septic shock with the use of norepinephrine/epinephrine and all conventional resuscitation measures (12).

In cases of suspected or confirmed cardiac dysfunction, dobutamine was prescribed (13).

We noted the presence or absence of initial shock on admission or during hospitalisation, and the use and duration of vasoactive drugs.

5.4.3. Pharmacological management :

All our patients received treatment in line with international recommendations and guidelines.

Treatments used :

▪ Anticoagulants :

Anticoagulation was either prophylactic or curative, in accordance with updated INEAS recommendations (depending on the presentation, clinical and biological form, the patient's background, and the presence or absence of a thromboembolic complication) (12).

▪ Corticosteroid therapy :

Based on dexamethasone at a dose of 8mg/d intravenously in a single dose for 10 days with no reduction (14).

▪ Antibiotic therapy :

Initially (at the start of the COVID 19 pandemic) it was systematic, but given the exceptional nature of bacterial co-infection during COVID, as described in the literature, antibiotic therapy was prescribed for patients presenting clinical, radiological or biological criteria suggesting co-infection or superinfection (15).

This initial antibiotic treatment was based on macrolides alone for five days or a combination of a beta-lactam or third-generation cephalosporin with a fluoroquinolone or macrolide.

In the event of suspected or confirmed superinfection, antibiotic therapy was initially empirical and then adapted to the microbiological data and ecology of the ward (if a nosocomial infection was suspected).

5.5 Evolution and complications 5.5.1- Short-term evolution

- NIV failure
- Use of a VMI
- Length of stay in intensive care.
- Duration of mechanical ventilation
- Mortality rate
- Time of death in relation to hospitalisation and causes of death.

5.5.2. Complications arising during hospitalisation

- Respiratory: ARDS...
- Cardiovascular: shock, thromboembolic complications
- Nosocomial infections.
- Other organ failure: renal.

5.6 Severity scores

5.6.1Severity scores at on admission

Initial severity on admission was expressed by scores:

➢ The Simplified Severity Index II :

The Simplified Severity Index II (IGSII score (16, 17)) is the most widely used severity score in intensive care in Europe. This system differs from others in that it is explicitly designed to predict in-hospital mortality, based on parameters present at admission or at the end of the first 24 hours of an ICU stay. **(Appendix 2)**

➢ Sequential Organ Failure Assessment Score:

Previously known as the Sepsis-related Organ Failure Assessment Score (SOFA Score (18)), currently used to assess the degree of organ dysfunction and clinical severity **(Appendix 3).**

6. Definitions

6.1 The definition of variables

6.1.1 Infection COVID 19

The diagnosis of a COVID 19 infection was made when :

- A positive test for SARS-CoV-2 viral RNA by RT-PCR from a nasopharyngeal wab.
- Strongly suggestive CT images.
- Positive COVID 19 IgM and/or IgG serology.
- Antigenic detection of COVID 19 using a rapid test.

6.1.2 A COVID 19 infection in its critical form :

According to the INEAS, it is defined by the presence of vital distress, shock, sepsis and/or organ failure and/or the need for invasive or non-invasive respiratory assistance with admission to an intensive care unit.

6.1.3 An infection nosocomial

This is an infection contracted in hospital. It was not present when the patient was admitted and occurs after more than 48 hours in a hospital establishment.

6.1.4 Hospital-acquired pneumonia

Nosocomial pneumopathies are grouped into mechanically ventilated pneumopathy and severe pneumonia, defined respectively as infections occurring after 48 hours of hospitalisation or mechanical ventilation (invasive or non-invasive) (19). The diagnostic criteria are clinical, biological and radiological (20).A VAP is said to be early if it occurs in less than 5 days. It is said to be late if it occurs within 5 days or more.

6.1.4. A urinary tract infection nosocomial

It is defined by the presence of at least one of the following signs: fever over 38°C, urinary urgency, urinary frequency, urinary burning, suprapubic pain in the absence of other causes (20). It can occur :

Without bladder catheterisation or other approaches to the urinary tract: leucocyturia ($\geq 10^4$ leucocytes/ml), a positive uroculture ($\geq 10^3$ micro-organisms/ml) and no more than two different micro-organisms.

- A positive uroculture ($\geq 10^5$ microorganisms/ml) and no more than two different microorganisms, with bladder catheterisation or other approaches to the urinary tract, in progress or within the previous seven days.

6.1.5. An infection linked to central catheters :

In the absence of bacteremia, the diagnosis of catheter-associated infection (CAI) is based on :

-A central venous catheter culture $\geq 10^3$ CFU/ml.

-And purulence from the catheter entry orifice or tunnelitis.

It is said to be bacteremic if it is associated with peripheral and central blood cultures positive for the same microorganism.

6.1.6. Bacteremia nosocomial

It is defined by the presence of at least one positive blood culture (associated with clinical signs suggestive of infection), except for the following saprophytic microorganisms (20) :

- A coagulase-negative staphylococcus
- A bacillus spp (except B. antracis)
- A corynebacterium spp
- A propionibacteruim spp
- Micrococcus spp or comparable pathogenic potential

It is necessary to have two blood cultures positive for the same germs, taken during different punctures, at different times, and within a short interval (a maximum of 48 hours is usually used).

6.1.7. Invasive candidiasis

Systemic or invasive candidiasis are defined as infections caused by yeasts belonging to the Candida group, which includes candidemiasis and deep visceral candidiasis (21).

6.1.8. Acute respiratory distress syndrome :

The definition of ARDS is based on the 4 so-called "Berlin criteria" proposed in 2012

- ARF that has been evolving for a week or less.
- This ARF is not entirely explained by heart failure.
- The presence of bilateral opacities on chest imaging.
- Hypoxaemia with a PaO2 / inspiratory oxygen fraction (FiO2) ratio <300 mmHg with a positive expiratory pressure set at 5 cmH2O or more.

Its severity depends on the PaO2/FiO2 ratio:

- Slight if 201≤ PaO2/FiO2 <300 mmHg.
- Moderate if 101≤ PaO2/FiO2 <200 mmHg.
- Severe if PaO2/FiO2 < 100 mmHg.

6.1.9 Acute renal failure

It is defined by the KDIGO (Kidney Disease Improving Global Outcomes) 2012 criteria by the presence of one of these criteria [14] :

- Increase in serum creatinine ≥0.3 mg/dl (≥26.5 μmol/l) within less than 48 hours.
- An increase in serum creatinine ≥1.5 times baseline levels within less than seven days.
- Diuresis <0.5 ml/kg/h for at least six hours.

There are three stages defined in the table below:

Table I: Stages of renal failure

Stadium	Creatinine	Diuresis
Stage I	1.5-1.9 times baseline creatinine Or ≥ 26.5 umol/l	<0.5ml/kg/h for 6-12h
Stage II	2-2.9 times baseline creatinine	<0.5ml/kg/h for ≥ 6-12h
Stage II	3 times or more baseline creatinine Or increase ≥ 353.6 umol/l Or extra-renal purification	< 0.3ml/kg/h for≥ 24h Or Anuria≥ 12h

6.1.10. Degree of radiological damage

Typical radiological involvement in COVID-19 pneumonia is defined by the presence of bilateral, multi-lobar, asymmetric, peripheral sub pleural ground-glass areas, often posterior and basal, on chest CT imaging (22). Parenchymal condensation may also be seen(23). Radiological involvement is estimated as a percentage of affected lung parenchyma and correlates with the clinical severity of the disease. It is progressive and may worsen as the disease progresses(24). The typical appearance of the progression over time of parenchymal damage associated with COVID is evidenced by the "crazy paving" appearance, which corresponds to the superimposition of areas of frosted glass and intra-lobular reticulations, as well as more or less retractile parenchymal condensations. Maximum CT involvement is observed at 10 days (22).

The Society of Thoracic Imaging (SIT) distinguishes 4 stages according to the degree of radiological involvement (22):

1- Minimal if less than 10% of the lung parenchyma is affected.

2- Moderate if parenchymal involvement between 10% and 25%.

3- Extensive if parenchymal involvement between 50% and 75%.

4- Critical if over 75%.

7. Analysis statistics

The data were collated and analysed using SPSS (Statistical Package for the Social Sciences) software version 24.0.

We calculated absolute frequencies and relative frequencies (percentages) for the qualitative variables. We calculated averages, medians and standard deviations, and determined extreme values for quantitative variables. We performed a bivariate analysis. For qualitative variables, we performed a Pearson chi-2 test. In the event of significance in the chi-2 test and the presence of at least one cell with a size of less than five, the two-tailed Fisher exact test was used. For quantitative variables, we performed a logistic regression with one variable at a time. In all statistical tests, the significance level was set at 0.05.

8. Search bibliography

Google was the most widely used search engine. The databases used to collect bibliographic data were mainly : Pubmed, Science Direct and Clinical Key. The keywords were consistent with those of the biomedical thesaurus i n French and English.

9. Ethical considerations

This was a descriptive study. Patients' anonymity was respected.The study was conducted in strict compliance with medical confidentiality. Clinical facts have been reported on a purely observational basis

RESULTS

1. Descriptive study

1.1. The population

During the 6-month study period, 47 of 251 patients admitted to intensive care were included in our study.

1.2. Age

The mean age was 61.4±12.7 years, with extremes ranging from 24 to 84 years (Figure 1).

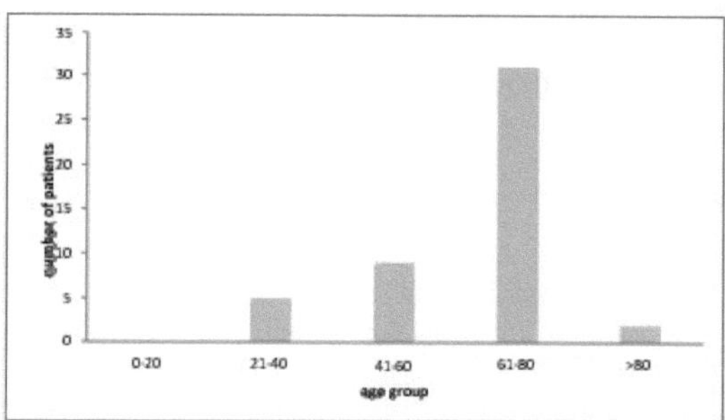

Figure 1: Breakdown of the population by age (years)

1.3. The genre

There was a predominance of males, with a sex ratio of 1.47 (Figure 2).

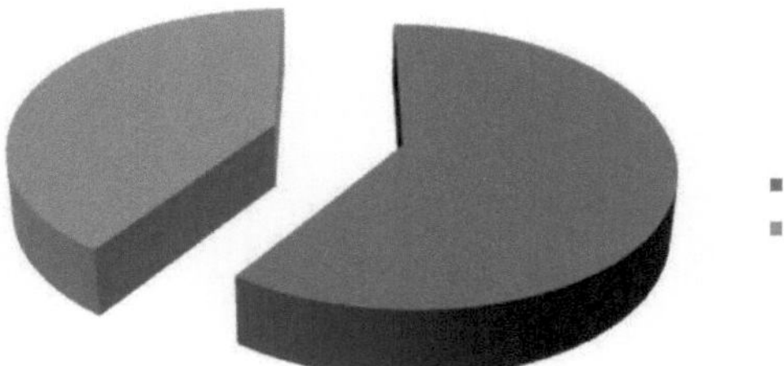

Figure 2: Breakdown of the population by gender

1.4. A history of pathological

Comorbidities were dominated by arterial hypertension, diabetes and dyslipidaemia. Ten patients, i.e. 21.7% of our population, were smokers. The average weight of our population was 84.6±21 Kg with an average BMI of 30.03±5.7. A detailed history is given in Table II.

Table II: Breakdown of the population according to antecedents

History	Number (n=47)	Percentage (%)
HTA	27	57.4
Diabetes	17	36.2
Dyslipidemia	9	21.4
Rhythm disorder	6	14.3
Chronic renal failure	5	11.8
COPD	3	6.4
Asthma	1	2.1
Active cancer	1	2.1

HTA: hypertension, COPD: chronic obstructive pulmonary bronchitis.

1.5. Gravity scores

The mean IGS II severity score was 32.8±11 (Figure 3).

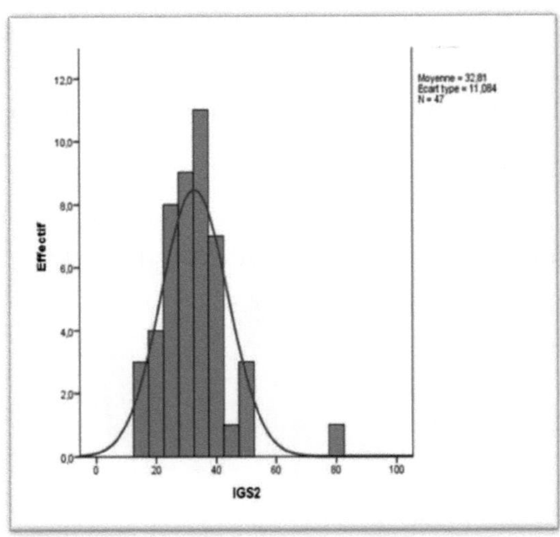

Figure 3: Distribution of the population according to IGSII score.

1.6. Clinical data

COVID-19 infection was confirmed either by a rapid test in 7 patients (12.7%) or by PCR-antiginemia in 32 patients (68%). The other patients were confirmed by radiological images.

The mean time to onset of symptoms on admission was 8.09±3 days [1-15]. All the population met thecriteria for the diagnosis of ARDS according to the Berlin definition. The classification of ARDS severity is detailed in Table III.

Table III: Distribution of our population according to the severity of ARDS.

ARDS	Number	Percentage (%)
Light	5	10.6
Moderate	24	51.1
Severe	17	38.3

ARDS: acute respiratory distress syndrome.

The various respiratory parameters recorded on admission are summarised in Table IV.

Table IV: Respiratory parameters on admission.

Respiratory parameters	MOY	AND	MINIMUM	MAXIMUM
Respiratory frequency	29.08	6.8	17	42
SpO2	91.04	8.42	60	100
FiO2	66.09	17	26	100

MOY: mean; SD: standard deviation; SpO2: peripheral O2 saturation; FiO2: fraction of inspired oxygen.

1.7. Biological data

On admission to the intensive care unit and during the first 24 hours, all patients underwent a blood count, haemostasis, renal and hepatic tests, blood ionogram, procalcitonin and troponin, the results of which are summarised in Table V.

Table V: Biological parameters on admission.

Balance sheet	ADMISSION	
	avg±ET	Min/Max
GB (elt/mm)3	10541±5283	3090/29030
Lymphocytes (elt/mm)3	961.9±485	240/2620
CRP	167.8±86	42/350
PCT	1.16±3,57	0.03/21.26
DDimére	3136±7637	190/44057
Fibrinogen	5.21±1.66	2.09/9.84
AST (IU/l)	60.5±75	17/447
ALT (IU/l)	153±180	9/334
LDH (IU/l)	624±326	155/1369
Troponin(ug/ml)	113±605	0.4/4031
Albumin levels	26.6±4.67	18/32
PaO2/FiO2	138±61.7	56/288

WBC: white blood cells, PCT: procalcitonin, LDH: lactic dehydrogenase, PaO2: arterial oxygen pressure, FiO2: fraction of inspired oxygen, PaO2/ FiO2: ratio, Avg: mean, SD: standard deviation, Min: minimum, Max: maximum.

1.8. Data scannographiques

Chest CT scans without contrast injection were performed in 45 patients (96%). The most common radiological abnormality was ground glass (95.6%), followed b y alveolar condensation (78.8%) and crazy paving (72.9%). Mean lung parenchymal involvement by COVID-19 was estimated at 67.5±17.3%. Figure 4 details the degree of CT lung involvement found on admission.

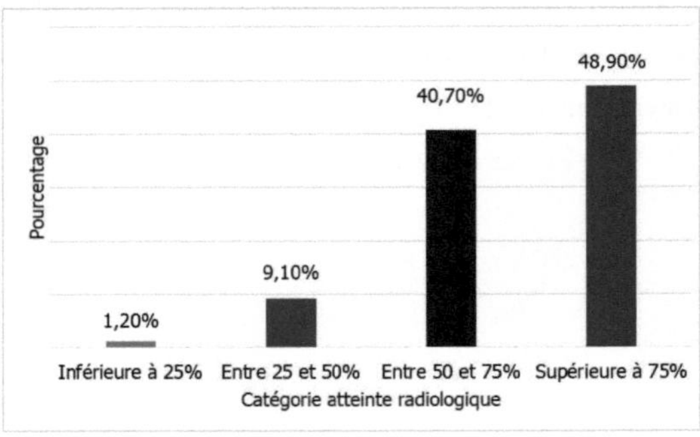

Figure 4: Distribution of the population according to the degree of scannographic lung damage.

1.9. Treatment options

1.9.1. Support ventilation

All patients required oxygen therapy to achieve SpO2 > 94%. The ventilatory supports used :

- High Flow Oxygen Therapy (HFO) :

Twenty-one patients (44.6%) benefited from OHD ventilatory support. The mean FiO2 was 74±22% [35-100] with a mean flow rate of 49.5±4.9L/min [35-60].

- Non-invasive ventilation (NIV) :

All patients using NIV with an average number of sessions per day of

2.57±0.65 [1-4] and a mean duration of 6.7±4.45 days [35-60]. The ventilatory parameters are detailed in table VI.

Table VI: Ventilatory parameters during non-invasive ventilation.

Ventilatory parameters	MOY	AND	MINIMUM	MAXIMUM
FiO2	72.2	2.2	17	42
PEP	8.85	1.16	6	12
AI	10.81	1.42	8	14

MOY: mean; SD: standard deviation; FiO2: fraction of inspired oxygen; PEP: positive expiratory pressure; AI: inspiratory aid.

- Invasive mechanical ventilation (IMV) :

Invasive mechanical ventilation was used in 13 patients (27.6%). The ventilatory mode used was controlled assisted ventilation in all patients, with a maximum FiO2 of 100%.

Patient ventilatory parameters and pressure monitoring are detailed in Table VII.

Table VII: Ventilatory parameters of patients undergoing invasive mechanical ventilation.

Ventilatory parameters	MOY	AND	MINIMUM	MAXIMUM
Tidal volume	430	62	330	560
PEP	9.68	1.8	6	14
Respiratory frequency	26	2.1	24	30
P.plat	27.2	3.7	21	36
P.mot	15.3	2.9	9	20

MOY: mean; SD: standard deviation; PEP: positive expiratory pressure; P. plat: plateau pressure; P.mot: motor pressure.

The mean duration of invasive mechanical ventilation was 10.53±8.1 [1-31].

1.9.2. Pharmacological management at on admission

1.9.2.1. Antibiotic therapy at on admission

Initial antibiotic therapy was indicated in all patients, with a 3[éme] generation cephalosporin in 74% of cases and amoxicillin-clavulanic acid in 24%.

1.9.2.2. Corticosteroid therapy

All patients were treated with dexamedasone-based corticosteroids at a dose of 8mg/d.

1.9.2.3. Sedation/curarisation

All mechanically ventilated patients, thirteen patients (27.7%), were recommended deep neurosedation and curarisation with a mean RASS score of -4.92±0.27 [-4,-5].

1.9.2.4. Prone position

The use of prone positions was indicated in 37 patients (78.7%). Twenty-five patients (53.1%) benefited from prone positions during spontaneous ventilation and twelve patients (25.5%) after invasive mechanical ventilation.

1.10. Evolving data

1.10.1. Complications

Complications encountered during a stay in intensive care are dominated by :

- Haemodynamic complications: Seventeen patients (36.1%) developed shock.
- Infectious complications: Sixteen patients (34%) developed a nosocomial infection during their stay. Bacterial origin was found in all cases. A nosocomial origin was found in 12 patients (25.5% of cases).
- Respiratory complications: We noted a respiratory complication in five patients of the barotrauma type. Subcutaneous emphysema was noted in 4 patients, pneumomediastinum in 4 patients and pneumothorax in one patient.
- A thrombo-embolic event: Eight patients developed a thrombo-embolic event. Five patients developed pulmonary embolism, two patients deep vein thrombosis and one patient arterial thrombosis.

1.10.2. Length of stay

The average length of stay in intensive care was 12.3±7.4 days, with a minimum of 1 day and a maximum of 35 days (Figure 5).

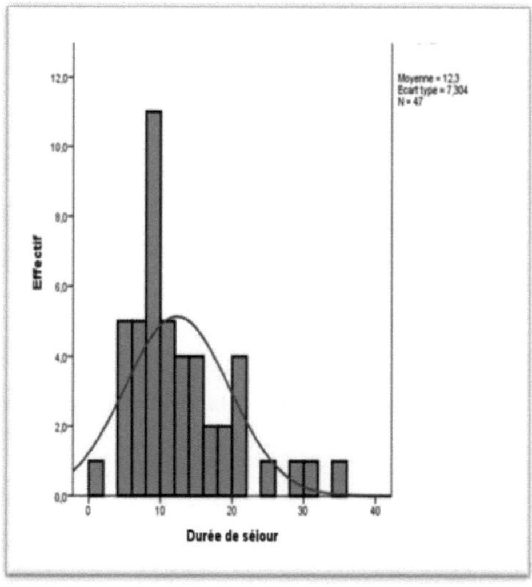

Figure 5: Breakdown of the population according to length of stay.

1.10.3. Mortality rate

Nineteen patients died during the study period. The mortality rate in the study population was 40.4%.

2. Univariate analytical study

2.1. Risk factors for NIV failure

2.1.1. Epidemiological data

Patients who failed NIV had a significantly higher mean age (68±6.3 vs 58±13.6; p=0.002).

ROC curve analysis showed that an age greater than 62 years was significantly correlated with a poor prognosis, with a sensitivity of 84%, a specificity of 55% and an AUC of 0.76 (Figure 6).

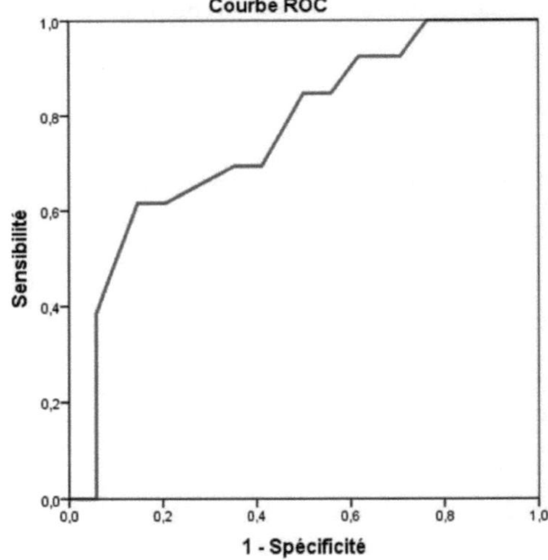

Figure 6: ROC curve illustrating the correlation between age and NIV failure.

Gender was not associated with the use of invasive mechanical ventilation in the population studied (p=0.58). Comorbidities were not associated with NIV failure in the population studied (Table VIII).

Table VIII: Univariate analysis of comorbidities.

History	Failure NAV (%)	Success NAV (%)	P
HTA	61	55.8	0.49
Diabetes	30.7	38.2	0.45
Dyslipidemia	16.6	23.3	0.49
Rhythm disorder	15.3	11.7	0.56
Respiratory history	23	11.7	0.41

HTA: high blood pressure.

BMI was higher in the NIV failure group without significant difference (30.5 vs 28.6; p=0.32).

2.1.2. Gravity scores

The mean IGSII score was higher in patients with NIV failure 38.1±14.1 vs 30.7±9.1 with p=0.039. ROC curve analysis showed that an IGS II score greater than 29 was significantly correlated with a poor prognosis, with a sensitivity of 84% and a specificity of 61%, with an AUC of 0.67 and p=0.03 (Figure 7).

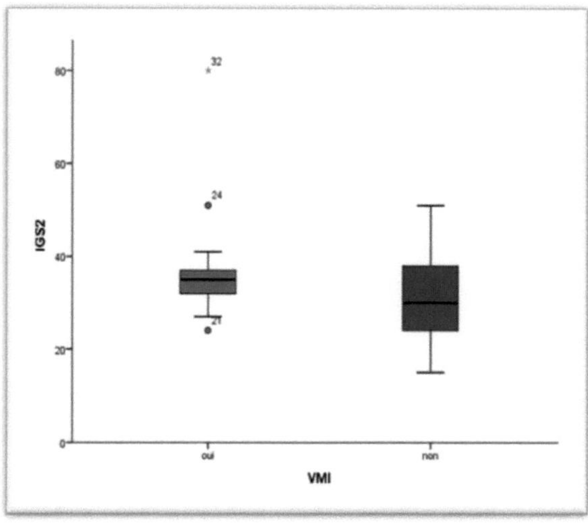

Figure 7: Comparison of IGSII averages.

2.1.3. Clinical data

Haemodynamic parameters were without difference between the 2 groups on admission. Severe acute respiratory distress syndrome was more common in patients with NIV failure (p=0.02), which explains the lower PaO2/FiO2 ratio (125±57 vs 143±63; p=0.04). The initial respiratory rate was higher in patients with NIV failure (33.7±5.8 vs 28.4±6.2; p=0.01) with a higher need for inspiratory support under NIV (11.5±1.1 vs 10.5±1.4; p=0.028). Table IX shows the clinical parameters collected on admission which correlate with mortality. The ROC curves for these parameters are shown in Figure 9--> 11.

Table IX: Clinical parameters correlated with mortality.

Parameters	Area under the curve	Sensitivity (%)	Specific (%)	P
EN > 26	0.73	84	52	0.028
AI > 11 On admission	0,67	69	41	0,021
PaO2/FiO2 < 105 On admission	0,59	70	54	0,05

FR: respiratory frequency; AI: inspiratory aid.

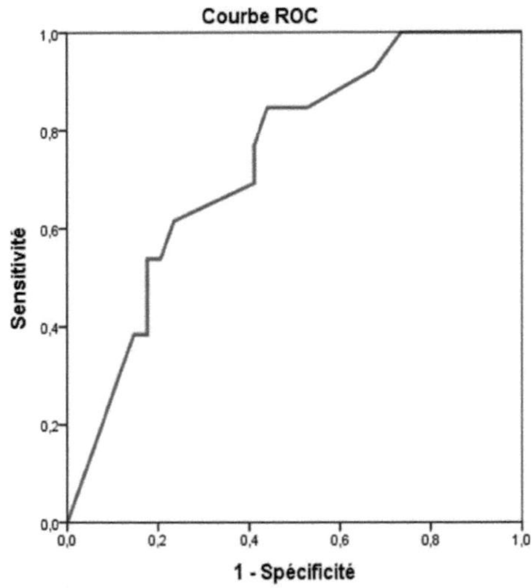

Figure 7: ROC curve illustrating the correlation between respiratory rate and NIV failure.

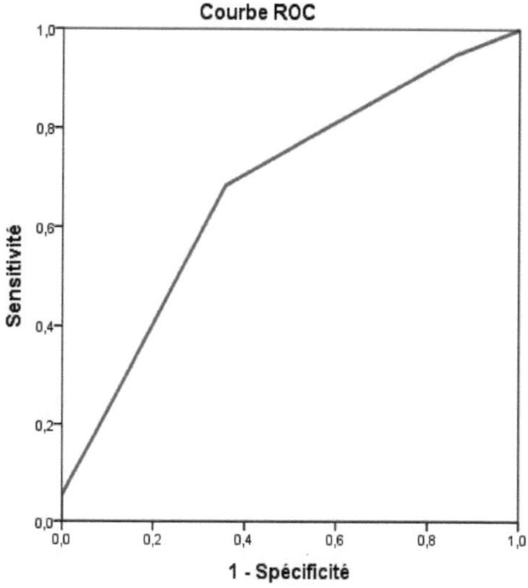

Figure 8: ROC curve illustrating the correlation between level of inspiratory support and NIV failure.

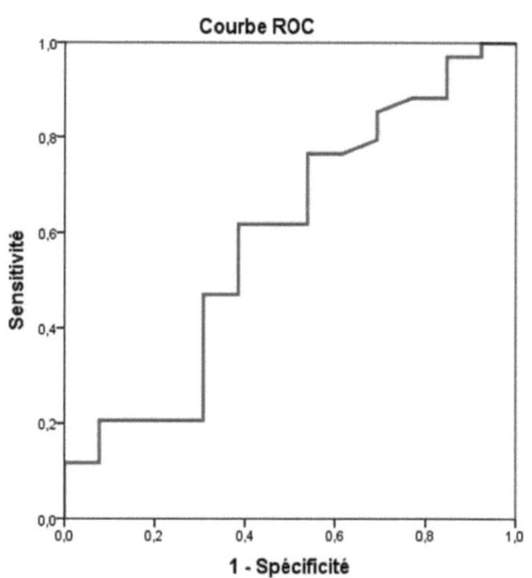

Figure 9: ROC curve illustrating the correlation between the PaO2/FiO2 ratio and NIV failure.

2.1.4. Biological data

Table X shows the biological parameters collected on admission and correlated with mortality. The ROC curves for these parameters are shown in Figures 12 and 13.

Table X: Paraclinical parameters correlated with mortality.

Biological parameters	Area under the curve	Sensitivity (%)	Specific (%)	P
CRP>150	0.68	69	44	0.05
Albumin < 25mg/l	0,85	80	40	0,003

Figure 10: ROC curve illustrating the correlation between CRP and NIV failure.

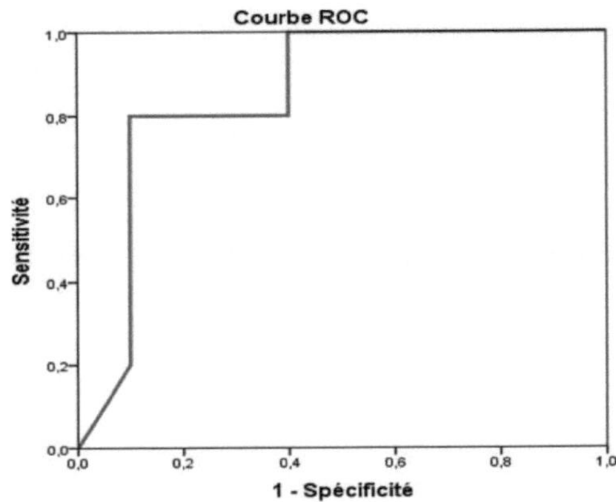

Figure 11: ROC curve illustrating the correlation between albumin and NIV failure.

2.1.5. Complications

The development of shock was a predictive factor for NIV failure (92.3% vs 14.7%; $p<10^{-3}$).

A finding of nosocomial infection in our population was more common in patients who used VMI ($p<10^{-3}$).

2.2. Risk factors for mortality

Those who died were older than those who survived (66.5 years vs 57.9 years; p=0.001). An age greater than 61 years is associated with a poor prognosis, with sensitivity of 89% and specificity of 57%, and an area under the curve of 0.75 (Figure 14).

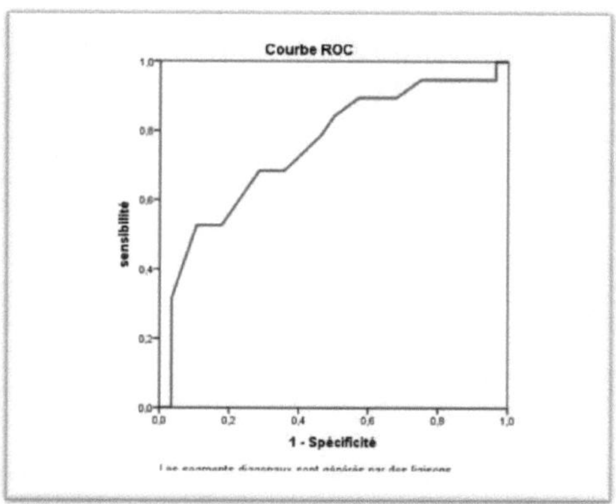

Figure 12: ROC curve illustrating the correlation between age and mortality.

An IGSII score greater than 28 points was predictive of mortality with a sensitivity of 89%, specificity of 53.6% and area under the curve of 0.78 (Figure 15).

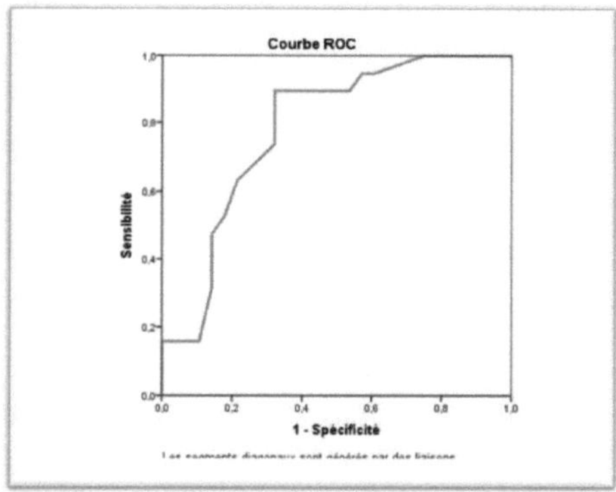

Figure 13: ROC curve illustrating the correlation between IGSII score and mortality.

The need for ventilatory support was more marked in decedents, as evidenced by a higher FiO2, AI under NIV and pep (Table XI).

Table XI: Ventilatory parameters correlated with mortality.

Ventilatory parameters	Area under the curve	Sensitivity (%)	Specific (%)	P
FiO2>60%	0.74	89	57	0.003
Inspiratory support > 11	0,67	68	45	0,025
PEP MAX > 9	0.73	78	50	0.004

FiO2: fraction of inspired oxygen; PEEP: positive expiratory pressure.

The use of invasive mechanical ventilation was predictive of mortality (68.5% vs 0%; p<10).[3]The presence of a pulmonary embolism was a factor in poor prognosis (36% vs. 10%; p=0.011).The development of shock and nosocomial infection were predictive of mortality failure ($p<10^{-3}$ and $p<10^{-3}$ respectively). The mean duration of was longer in deceased patients, with a significant difference (14.2±7.1 vs 8±7.8; p=0.007).

3. Multi-varied analytical study

All the factors correlated with prognosis identified in the univariate analysis were incorporated into multivariate analysis models constructed using the top-down stepwise method. The least significant factor was removed from the model until all factors were significant.Finally, the independent factors correlated with NIV failure were a respiratory rate greater than 25 cpm and inspiratory support greater than 11 cmH2O.

Table XII: Independent factors predictive of NIV failure.

Factors	P	OR	Minimum	Maximum
FR > 25 cpm	0,028	4,54	3,7	44,3
AI > 11 cm H2O	0,021	32,2	22,5	80,7

DISCUSSION

1. Main results

We conducted a retrospective study of 47 patients admitted to intensive care with severe forms of confirmed SARS-CoV-2 infection. The mean age was 61.4±12.7 years with a sex ratio of 1.47. Comorbidities were dominated by arterial hypertension, diabetes and dyslipidaemia. Ten patients, i.e. 21.7% of our population, were smokers. The mean BMI was 30.03±5.7. The mean IGS II severity score was 32.8±11. COVID-19 infection was confirmed either by a rapid test in 7 patients (12.7%) or by PCR-antiginemia in 32 patients (68%). The other patients were confirmed by radiological images. The mean time to onset of symptoms on admission was 8.09±3 days [1-15].The clinical picture on admission consisted mainly of polypnoea, with a mean respiratory rate of 29.08±6.8 cycles/min. Almost all (94%) of the patients had ARDS. ARDS was mild in 10.6% of cases, moderate in 51.1% and severe in 38.3%. All patients required oxygen therapy to achieve SpO2 > 94%. Twenty-one patients (44.6%) benefited from OHD-type ventilatory support. The mean FiO2 was 74±22% [35-100] with a mean flow rate of 49.5±4.9L/min [35-60]. All patients had recourse to NIV with a mean number of sessions per day of 2.57±0.65 [1-4] and a mean duration of 6.7±4.45 days [35-60]. The mean PaO2/FiO2 ratio on admission was 138±61.7mmHg. The mortality rate was 40.4%.The independent factors for NIV failure in univariate analysis in our study were: age over 62 years, IGSII score over 29, severe ARDS with a PaO2/FiO2 ratio below 105 mmHg, need for inspiratory support over 11, respiratory rate on admission over 26 cycles/min, CRP level over 150 mg/l, albumin level below 25, development of shock and nosocomial infection.The independent factors for mortality in univariate analysis in our study were: age greater than 61 years, IGS II score greater than 28, ventilatory parameters under NIV: FiO2>60%, inspiratory aid greater than 11 and positive expiratory pressure greater than 9, recourse to invasive mechanical ventilation, development of shock and occurrence of nosocomial infection.

Weak points

This study has several limitations:

- This was a retrospective observational study.

- A small number of patients were already receiving NIV, which did not allow us to draw too many conclusions in this respect.

• The vaccination status of patients was not taken into account in this study.

2. Incidence and epidemiology

✚ Incidence

The rate of admission to intensive care during the COVID-19 pandemic varied from one country to another and from one hospital centre to another. It was 28.8% in a hospital in Dubai (25) and 5.8% in Madrid (26). The national rate was estimated at 27.16% (27).

The admission rate to our intensive care unit was 31%.

✚ Age and sex

An average age of 63 years has been reported in Italy (28) and in a meta-analysis of intensive care units in France, Switzerland and Belgium (29). An average age of 70 has been reported in Washington (30).Our population was similar to that hospitalised in Sfax (62.4 years) (31) and La Rabta (63 years) (32).

In our study, the gender ratio was 1.32. This predominance of males with different sex ratios has been reported in the majority of studies in different countries (29).

✚ Comorbidities

➢ Obesity has been correlated with the development of severe forms of COVID-19, but its direct impact on mortality remains unclear.

In a meta-analysis by Huang et al (33) of over 30 studies, obesity was associated with a high risk of developing a severe form of the disease with an Odds Ratio (OR) of 1.76, an increased risk of admission to intensive care with an OR of 2.19 and an increased risk of recourse to invasive mechanical ventilation and therefore of death with an OR=1.37. In the study by Ejaz et al (34) 68.6% of obese patients in intensive care required invasive mechanical ventilation.

➢ Hypertension and diabetes were the two most frequently reported comorbidities in the literature, with percentages varying from one study to another.

Table XII below summarises the prevalence of hypertension and diabetes by study country.

Table XII: Prevalence of hypertension and diabetes by country

Study [Reference]	Country	HTA (%)	Diabetes (%)
Grasselli et al (35)	Lombardy, Italy	41,2	12,9
Palaiodimos et al (36)	New York, United States	76	39,5
Borobia et al (37)	Madrid, Spain	52	28
Pederson et al (38)	Denmark	56	13
Bahloul et al (31)	Sfax, Tunisia	50	46

HTA: high blood pressure

Gravity scores

Calculating severity scores on admission to the intensive care unit is an effective tool for estimating patient severity and assessing prognosis (39). They remain applicable for patients with severe SARS-CoV-2 infection.

➢ **Simplified Severity Index (SSI):** The mean SSI score for our patients was 32.8±11. This value is close to that found in a European meta-analysis (40). Lazero et al (41) reported a mean IGS score of 68.5 in deceased COVID-19 patients. This score was significantly associated with high mortality.

3. Clinical pictures

➢ The average duration of onset of symptoms in our population was 8.09±3 days. This value is similar to that reported in Italy (35) and China (42).

➢ A positive diagnosis of SARS-CoV-2 infection was based on a positive RT-PCR obtained from a nasopharyngeal swab. This method has a high specificity and a sensitivity of between 60 and 80%. (43). Other diagnostic methods have been validated, namely the rapid antigen test, which has a high positive predictive value, with a result obtained after 20 minutes.

➢ All our patients had ARDS. The mean PaO2/FiO2 ratio on admission to intensive care was 138±61mmHg. This value is lower than that recorded in Sfax (median PaO2/FiO2 150mmHg) (31). The prevalence of ARDS differs from one study to another, and was 100% in a study conducted in Washington in the United States, with a median PaO2/FiO2 ratio of 169mmHg (30). In a Chinese meta-analysis, the prevalence of ARDS was 63%, with a median PaO2/FiO2 ratio of 100mmHg (42).

➢ The mean lymphocyte count was 961elt/mm^3 . The mean white blood cell count on admission to intensive care was 10541elt/mm^3 . The mean CRP level was 167 mg/l. These findings are consistent with those of several studies in different countries (32,39).

4. Ventilatory management

➢ **High-flow oxygen therapy:** delivers an oxygen flow of up to 60 L/min via a nasal cannula, a reduced dead space and a PEEP of up to 5 mmHg, in addition to humidified mucociliary clearance (44).

This technique has gained interest because it is well tolerated in extremely hypoxic patients.

➢ **Non-invasive ventilation (VS-AI-PEEP mode):** NIV improves alveolar ventilation, reduces capnia and increases PaO2, mainly due to the significant PEEP effect. It is still of interest in hypercapnic patients or if there is associated cardiac decompensation (44).

The indications for non-invasive ventilation remain debated, the dilemma being the fear of delaying inevitable intubation *and therefore increasing mortality. Several protocols have been proposed for choosing ventilatory support according to the PaO2/FiO2 ratio and the clinical presentation (respiratory frequency, use of accessory respiratory muscles) (45).

In a review and meta-analysis of 25 RCTs involving 3804 patients, Ferreyro BL et al. reported the evidence for the efficacy of NIV compared with conventional oxygen therapy in the management of ARF (46). In a multi-centre randomised trial including 4 intensive care units and 110 patients in Italy (The HENIVOT study), which compared patients who received NIV versus those who received NIV, the results were as follows The authors report a significantly higher rate of intubation in the OHD group. However, the mortality rate was the same in both groups (47). Table XIII below summarises the rate of use of non-invasive ventilation in various countries.

Table XIII: Non-invasive ventilation by country of study.

Study [Reference]	Country	NAV (%)	OHD (%)
Grasselli et al [46]	Lombardy, Italy	8,77	-
Arentez et al [48]	Washington, United States	19	17,8
Serafim et al [51]	Meta analysis	25,5	20,5
Gupta et al [71]	United States	18,5	1,2
Yuang et al [53]	China	56	33
Saida et al [62]	Sousse, Tunisia	40	-
Bahloul et al [49]	Sfax Tunisia	50	31

➢ **Invasive mechanical ventilation:** oro-tracheal intubation is a cornerstone of the management of severe forms of SARS-CoV-2 infection. At the start of the pandemic, it was the main means of ventilation. As the pandemic progressed, this rate fell. We cite the example of a meta-analysis, where the rate of intubated patients was 58%(29) and a rate of 21% in Egypt (49).

Our strategy during the study period was to resort to invasive mechanical ventilation if non-invasive means failed, hemodynamic instability was present or there was an imminent risk of cardio respiratory arrest.All our patients were sedated with Midazolam and Fentanyl and curarised with Cisatracurium with a target SpO2 between 88 and 92%. We followed the strategy of protective ventilation with the main objective of a plateau pressure of less than 30cmH2O. Post-intubation DV was performed from a PaO2/FiO2 ratio of less than 150mmHg.

Table IVX summarises the different ventilatory parameters recorded on the first day of intubation.

Table XIV: Ventilatory parameters on the first day of invasive ventilation

Ventilatory parameter	Grasselli et al (50)	ICU covid group N (51)	Mitral et al (52)
Tidal volume (ml)	5.6-7.6 Ml/kg	6ml/Kg	400
PEEP (cmH2O)	9-16	12	12
Plateau pressure (cmH2O)	20.5-30	24	29
Static compliance (cmH2O)	24-49	33	35

PEEP: positive expiratory pressure

5. Complications

➢ Hospital-acquired infections

The rate of nosocomial infections is close to that reported by Badri et al (53) (40.7%). However, our results run counter to those reported in the same study, where catheter-related infection was the most frequent infection.

➢ Acute renal failure

The onset of acute renal failure in COVID-19 is multi-factorial. It is secondary to a direct action of the virus, thrombi secondary to endothelitis and an increase in pro-inflammatory cytokines (54). Indirect mechanisms leading to this complication are hypovolaemia and haemodynamic instability, in addition to iatrogenic factors (medical treatment, iodinated contrast products). The incidence of renal failure varies from one series to another. For example, the prevalence of acute renal failure was 19% in the United States (30) and 28% in a meta-analysis (31).

➢ **Other complications.**

Pulmonary embolism was diagnosed in 9% of patients in a meta-analysis including 4244 patients (9%). However, this figure is underestimated because angiography was not systematically performed.

- **Length of stay in intensive care :**

The length of stay in our intensive care unit was 12.3 days, with extremes of 1 and 35 days.

Our results are similar to those reported in Italy (12 days) (35) but lower than those reported in China (7 days) (42)]. This difference may be explained by the inhomogeneity of the population admitted to intensive care from one country to another.

- **In-hospital mortality :**

The mortality rate in our intensive care unit was 40.4%.

It was slightly lower than that reported in a study carried out in the intensive care unit at La Rabta (59%) (32).Table XV below summarises the mortality rates recorded in intensive care in various studies.

Table XV: Mortality in intensive care units in some published studies

Study [Reference]	Country	Mortality rate (%)
Grassalli et al (35)	Italy	53,4
Yang et al (42)	China	61,5
Gupta et al (48)	United States	39,5
Saida et al (40)	Tunisia (Sousse)	70
Armstrong et al (55)	Great Britain	41,6
Bahloul et al (31)	Tunisia (Sfax)	49

6. Factors linked to NAV failure

Prior to the COVID-19 pandemic, the use of non-invasive ventilation in hypoxaemic ARF was long debated (56). This strategy evolved progressively during the COVID-19 epidemic, depending on several factors: fear (57), availability of ventilators and intensive care beds, and understanding of the pathophysiology of COVID-19. In large cohorts describing the outcome of critically ill COVID-19 patients, the NIV failure rate is estimated to be between 11% and 80%(58).In an analysis of 85 observational studies and two RCTs, Weerakkody et al. reported a success rate of 61% in 12633 patients with severe COVID-19 treated with NIV (59). Although the predictors of NIRS failure may overlap as described by Liu et al (62), other studies suggest that they differ depending on the strategy used (60).

- A higher respiratory rate was significantly correlated with NIV failure in the present study. Respiratory rate has been suggested as a relevant parameter in the follow-up of ARF patients on NIPPV(84). The results of several studies of COVID-19 patients have also identified respiratory rate as a predictor of failure. In fact, polypnoea and high-volume breathing aggravate damage to an already damaged lung (61).

- In a study conducted in Zaghouan including 170 patients on the factors associated with failure of non-invasive ventilation in covid-19 patients, it was demonstrated that failure was significantly associated with a severe form of ARDS, an extent of parenchymal damage greater than 75%, non-adherence to the prone position and bacterial superinfection. Multivariate analysis concluded that two independent factors predicted failure: severe ARDS and bacterial superinfection, with ORs equal to 11 [3.6-33]; $p<0.05$ and 1.64 [0.7-3.9]; $p=0.03$ respectively (62).

- Bertaina et al in a retrospective study including 1933 patients identified the following factors: age, hypertension, SpO2 at AA less than 92%, lymphopenia and the use of antibiotics are predictive factors of NIV failure (63).

- Girault et al demonstrated that age, diabetes, immunosuppression, severity of obesity and severe ARDS were correlated with intubation and NIV failure (64).

In our population, the independent factors for NIV failure in the univariate analysis in our study were: age greater than 62 years, an IGSII score greater than 29, severe ARDS with a PaO2/FiO2 ratio less than 105 mmHg, a need for inspiratory support greater than 11, a respiratory rate on admission greater than 26 cycles/min, a CRP level greater than 150 mg/l, an albumin level less than 25, the development of shock and a nosocomial

infection.

7. Factors linked to mortality

In the literature, the factors linked to mortality vary from one study to another. For example :

- in the study by Gassalli et al (35) in the Lambardie region of Italy, which experienced one of the most severe waves in Europe, mortality was linked to age, gender male, the low PaO2/FiO2 ratio on admission and the need for a higher FiO2 and PEEP. In this study, the PaO2/FiO2 ratio was less than 103mmHg in 461 of the patients who died and between 103 and 144mmHg in 384 of them. FiO2 was greater than 82% in 501 of the patients who died and PEEP was greater than 12cmH2O in 814 of the patients who did not survive (35).

- In a meta-analysis in China, mortality was linked to age, the low PaO2/FiO2 ratio (100mmHg in surviving patients versus 62.5mmHg in those who died) andthe need forinvasivemechanical ventilation(42).

- In the US study by Gupta et al (48), mortality was associated with age, male gender, high BMI and a PaO2/FiO2 ratio of less than 100mmHg.

- In Tunisia, in the Sfax intensive care unit, the independent factors associated with mortality were the use of invasive ventilation and the occurrence of acute renal failure (65). In another study conducted in the La Rabta intensive care unit, the independent mortality factors identified were a CRP greater than 139.7mg/l, the onset of shock and a history of arterial hypertension (32).

The independent factors for mortality in univariate analysis in our study were: age greater than 61 years, IGS II score greater than 28, ventilatory parameters under NIV: FiO2>60%, inspiratory aid greater than 11 and positive expiratory pressure greater than 9, recourse to invasive mechanical ventilation, development of shock and occurrence of nosocomial infection.

CONCLUSION

Covid-19 is a new and emerging disease, characterised by an epidemiological evolution in successive waves. This was explained by the mutagenic power of the virus, creating different epidemiological profiles from one country to another.
with different clinical presentations.

Symptoms can range from mild forms with a simple cough and flu-like symptoms, to severe forms with acute respiratory failure that can progress to acute respiratory distress syndrome. These severe forms require intensive care, with frequent recourse to mechanical ventilation.

Initially, in the absence of a well-defined consensus and the availability of different ventilation devices, ventilatory management differed from one team to another. Some teams recommended invasive mechanical ventilation from the outset, to limit the risk of aerosolisation and contamination. Others opted for non-invasive ventilation as a first-line treatment, with invasive ventilation being used if this failed.

Currently, for most teams, non-invasive ventilation remains the reference ventilatory technique, in particular the SV-AI-PEP mode (5). Its aim is to avoid recourse to invasive mechanical ventilation, which is associated with a high mortality rate (3). A better understanding of the factors leading to NIV failure could enable intensive care units to establish dynamic management of this serious condition, in order to guarantee optimal, appropriate care.

The aim of our study was to describe the epidemiological, clinical, radiological and therapeutic characteristics, as well as the ventilatory strategy, of patients hospitalised with severe COVID19 pneumonia, and to identify factors predictive of NIV failure.

We conducted a descriptive, retrospective, monocentric study in the emergency department and medical intensive care unit of the Habib Thameur Hospital in Tunis, over a period from 07/07/2020 to 31/12/2020. We included patients with a COVID 19 infection in its critical form according to the INEAS definition (April 2021) and hospitalised for more than 48 hours with an age greater than 18 years and with a need for non-invasive ventilatory support. We did not include patients admitted for non-critical COVID 19 with a length of stay of less than 48 hours. The primary outcome was failure of NIV and use of invasive mechanical ventilation. The secondary outcome was mortality.During the 6-month study period, 47 of 251 patients admitted to intensive care were included in our study. The mean age was 61.4±12.7

years with extremes ranging from 24 to 84 years with a male predominance and a sex ratio of 1.47.Comorbidities were dominated by arterial hypertension, diabetes and dyslipidaemia. Ten patients, i.e. 21.7% of our population, were smokers. The average weight of our population was 84.6 ± 21 kg, with an average BMI of 30.03 ± 5.7. The mean IGS II severity score was 32.8±11. Infection with COVID-19 was confirmed either by a rapid test in 7 patients (12.7%) or by antiginemia PCR in 32 patients (68%). The other patients were confirmed by radiological images.The mean time to onset of symptoms on admission was 8.09±3 days [1-15]. The entire population met the criteria for a diagnosis of ARDS according to the Berlin definition. The mean PaO2/FiO2 ratio was 138±61.7 mm Hg with extremes of 56 and 288 mm Hg. Biologically, the mean WBC count was 10541±5283 elt/mm^3 and the mean lymphocyte count was 961.9±485 elt/mm .^{3}

Chest CT scans without contrast injection were performed in 45 patients (96%). The most common radiological abnormality was ground glass (95.6%), followed by alveolar condensation (78.8%) and crazy paving (72.9%).

Mean lung parenchymal involvement by COVID-19 was estimated at 67.5±17.3%. All patients required oxygen therapy to achieve SpO2 > 94%.

Twenty-one patients (44.6%) received OHD ventilatory support. The mean FiO2 was 74±22% [35-100] with a mean flow rate of 49.5±4.9L/min [35-60]. All patients using NIV with an average number of sessions per day of

2.57±0.65 [1-4] and a mean duration of 6.7±4.45 days [35-60]. Invasive mechanical ventilation was used in 13 patients (27.6%). The ventilatory mode used was controlled assisted ventilation in all patients with a maximum of FiO2 at 100%. The mean duration of invasive mechanical ventilation was 10.53±8.1 [1- 31].

Initial antibiotic therapy was indicated in all patients, with a 3^{éme} generation cephalosporin in 74% of cases and amoxicillin-clavulanic acid in 24%. All patients were treated with dexamedasone-based corticosteroids at a dose of 8mg/d. All mechanically ventilated patients, thirteen patients (27.7%), were recommended deep neurosedation and curarisation with a mean RASS score of -4.92±0.27 [-4,-5].

The use of prone positions was indicated in 37 patients (78.7%). Twenty-five patients (53.1%) benefited from prone positions during spontaneous ventilation and twelve patients (25.5%) after invasive mechanical ventilation. Seventeen patients (36.1%) developed shock. Sixteen patients (34%) developed a nosocomial infection during their stay. Bacterial origin was found in all cases. A nosocomial origin was found in 12 patients (25.5% of cases). We noted a respiratory complication in five patients of the barotrauma type. Subcutaneous emphysema was noted in 4 patients, pneumomediastinum in 4 patients and pneumothorax in one patient. Eight patients developed thromboembolic events. Five patients developed pulmonary embolism, two patients deep vein thrombosis and one patient arterial thrombosis. The mortality rate in the population studied was 40.4%, with an average length of stay in intensive care of 12.3±7.4 days, with a minimum of 1 day and a maximum of 35 days.

In univariate analysis, the risk factors for NIV failure were age greater than 62 years (p=0.002), an IGSII score greater than 29 points (p=0.03), the presence of ARDS (p=0.02), respiratory rate > 26c/min (p=0.028), inspiratory support > 11 (p=0.021), PaO2/FiO2 ratio < 105 (p=0.05), CRP > 150, albumin <25 and shock (p<10).$^{-3}$

The risk factors for failure to achieve mortality were: age greater than 61 years (p=0.001), an IGSII> 28 points, an inspired O2 fraction >60% (p=0.003), an inspiratory aid greater than 11 (p=0.025), a positive expiratory pressure greater than 9 (p=0.004), recourse to invasive mechanical ventilation (p<10^{-3}), the presence of a pulmonary embolism (p=0.01), the development of a state of shock (p<10^{-3}) and a nosocomial infection (p<10).$^{-3}$

At the end of our study, we were able to identify factors predictive of NIV failure and the need for invasive ventilatory support. We also identified poor prognostic factors associated with in-hospital mortality. This would make it possible, in the event of new waves, to triage patients and ensure better management of intensive care units, and hence optimal care.

REFERENCES

1. situations_particulieres_25_mars.pdf [Internet]. [cited 6 Apr 2023]. Available from: https://www.ineas.tn/sites/default/files//rapport-publication/situations_particulieres_25_mars.pdf

2. Broadley T, Burrell A, Carson G, Citarella BW, Dunning J, Elotmani L, et al. ISARIC COVID-19 Clinical Data Report issued: 15 December 2021.

3. Wiersinga WJ, Rhodes A, Cheng AC, Peacock SJ, Prescott HC. Pathophysiology, Transmission, Diagnosis, and Treatment of Coronavirus Disease 2019 (COVID-19): A Review. JAMA. August 25, 2020;324(8):782-93.

4. Liu L, Xie J, Wu W, Chen H, Li S, He H, et al. A simple nomogram for predicting failure of non-invasive respiratory strategies in adults with COVID-19: a retrospective multicentre study. Lancet Digit Health. March 2021;3(3):e166-74.

5. Jog S, Zirpe K, Dixit S, Godavarthy P, Shahane M, Kadapatti K, et al. Noninvasive Respiratory Assist Devices in the Management of COVID-19-related Hypoxic Respiratory Failure: Pune ISCCM COVID-19 ARDS Study Consortium (PICASo). Indian J Crit Care Med Peer-Rev Off Publ Indian Soc Crit Care Med. Jul 2022;26(7):791-7.

6. Tobin MJ. The criteria used to justify endotracheal intubation of patients with COVID-19 are worrisome. Can J Anaesth J Can Anesth. Feb 2021;68(2):258-9.

7. Boscolo A, Pasin L, Sella N, Pretto C, Tocco M, Tamburini E, et al. Outcomes of COVID-19 patients intubated after failure of non-invasive ventilation: a multicenter observational study. Sci Rep [Internet]. 6 Sep 2021 [cited 6 Apr 2023];11:17730. Available from: https://www.ncbi.nlm.nih.gov/pmc/articles/PMC8421335/

8. Hakim R, Watanabe-Tejada L, Sukhal S, Tulaimat A. Acute respiratory failure in randomized trials of noninvasive respiratory support: A systematic review of definitions, patient characteristics, and criteria for intubation. J Crit Care. June 2020;57:141-7.

9. Lodé B, Jalaber C, Orcel T, Morcet-Delattre T, Crespin N, Voisin S, et al. Imaging of COVID-19 pneumonia. J Imag Diagn Interv. Sept 2020;3(4):249-58.

10. on behalf of the European Society of Radiology (ESR) and the European Society of Thoracic Imaging (ESTI), Revel MP, Parkar AP, Prosch H, Silva M, Sverzellati N, et al. COVID-19 patients and the radiology department - advice from the European Society of

Radiology (ESR) and the European Society of Thoracic Imaging (ESTI). Eur Radiol. Sept 2020;30(9):4903-9.

11. Attaway AH, Scheraga RG, Bhimraj A, Biehl M, Hatipoğlu U. Severe covid-19 pneumonia: pathogenesis and clinical management. BMJ. 10 March 2021;n436.

12. Evolutionary guidelines for the clinical management of COVID-19 [Internet]. WHO; 2021.Available at: https://apps.who.int/iris/bitstream/handle/10665/352279/WHO-2019-nCoV-clinical-2021.2- fre.pdf

13. The INEAS Guides: GUIDE TO THE SUSPECTED PATIENT'S PATHWAY OR CONFIRMED COVID-19. [Internet]. 2021. Available on: https://www.ineas.tn/sites/default/files/gpc_covid_19_version_11_mai_2021.pdf

14. Wagner C, Griesel M, Mikolajewska A, Mueller A, Nothacker M, Kley K, et al. Systemic corticosteroids for the treatment of COVID-19. Cochrane Haematology Group, editor. Cochrane Database Syst Rev [Internet]. 16 Aug 2021 [cited 19 Dec 2022];2021(8). Disponible sur: http://doi.wiley.com/10.1002/14651858.CD014963

15. Langford BJ, So M, Raybardhan S, Leung V, Soucy JPR, Westwood D, et al. Antibiotic prescribing in patients with COVID-19: rapid review and meta-analysis. Clin Microbiol Infect. Apr 2021;27(4):520-31.

16. Godinjak AG. Predictive value of SAPS II and APACHE II scoring systems for patient outcome in medical intensive care unit. Acta Medica Acad. 6 Dec 2016;45(2):89-95.

17. Naved SA, Siddiqui S, Khan FH. APACHE-II score correlation with mortality and length of stay in an intensive care unit. J Coll Physicians Surg--Pak JCPSP. Jan 2011;21(1):4-8.

18. Vincent JL, Moreno R, Takala J, Willatts S, De Mendonça A, Bruining H, et al. The SOFA (Sepsis-related Organ Failure Assessment) score to describe organ dysfunction/failure: On behalf of the Working Group on Sepsis-Related Problems of the European Society of Intensive Care Medicine (see contributors to the project in the appendix). Intensive Care Med. July 1996;22(7):707-10.

19. Leone M, Bouadma L, Bouhemad B, Brissaud O, Dauger S, Gibot S, et al. Pneumonia associated with resuscitation care. Anesth Réanimation. sept 2018;4(5):421-41.

20. 5th Consensus Conference. Réanimation. Feb 2010;19(1):4-14.

21. Eggimann P, Pittet D. Candidoses en réanimationCandidiasis and intensive care patients.

Réanimation. May 2002;11(3):209-21.

22. Chest CT in COVID-19 pneumonia: A review of current knowledge - PubMed [Internet]. [cited 6 Apr 2023]. Available from: https://pubmed.ncbi.nlm.nih.gov/32571748/

23. Sun Z, Zhang N, Li Y, Xu X. A systematic review of chest imaging findings in COVID-19. Quant Imaging Med Surg. May 2020;10(5):1058-79.

24. Thoracic imaging in COVID-19 - PubMed [Internet]. [cited 6 Apr 2023]. Available from: https://pubmed.ncbi.nlm.nih.gov/32737043/

25. Iy H, My H, H H, Kb N, A S, S H. The inflammatory biomarkers profile of hospitalized patients with COVID-19 and its association with patient's outcome: A single centered study. PloS One [Internet]. 12 Feb 2021 [cited 29 Apr 2023];16(12). Available from: https://pubmed.ncbi.nlm.nih.gov/34855832/

26. Jiménez E, Fontán-Vela M, Valencia J, Fernandez-Jimenez I, Álvaro-Alonso EA, Izquierdo-García E, et al. Characteristics, complications and outcomes among 1549 patients hospitalised with COVID-19 in a secondary hospital in Madrid, Spain: a retrospective case series study. BMJ Open. 10 Nov 2020;10(11):e042398.

27. Harizi C, Cherif I, Najar N, Osman M, Mallekh R, Ayed OB, et al. Characteristics and prognostic factors of COVID-19 among infected cases: a nationwide Tunisian analysis. BMC Infect Dis. 3 Feb 2021;21(1):140.

28. Grasselli G, Greco M, Zanella A, Albano G, Antonelli M, Bellani G, et al. Risk Factors Associated With Mortality Among Patients With COVID-19 in Intensive Care Units in Lombardy, Italy. JAMA Intern Med. 1 Oct 2020;180(10):1345-55.

29. Serafim RB, Póvoa P, Souza-Dantas V, Kalil AC, Salluh JIF. Clinical course and outcomes of critically ill patients with COVID-19 infection: a systematic review. Clin Microbiol Infect [Internet]. Jan 2021 [cited 6 Dec 2022];27(1):47-54. Available from: https://linkinghub.elsevier.com/retrieve/pii/S1198743X20306480

30. Characteristics and Outcomes of 21 Critically Ill Patients With COVID-19 in Washington State. 2020;3.

31. Bahloul M, Kharrat S, Chtara K, Hafdhi M, Turki O, Baccouche N, et al. Clinical characteristics and outcomes of critically ill COVID-19 patients in Sfax, Tunisia. Acute Crit Care [Internet]. 28 Feb 2022 [cited 6 Dec 2022];37(1):84-93. Available from: http://accjournal.org/journal/view.php?doi=10.4266/acc.2021.00129

32. Emna ABID.pdf.

33. Huang Y, Lu Y, Huang YM, Wang M, Ling W, Sui Y, et al. Obesity in patients with COVID-19: a systematic review and meta-analysis. Metabolism [Internet]. Dec 2020 [cited 6 Dec 2022];113:154378. Available at: https://linkinghub.elsevier.com/retrieve/pii/S0026049520302420

34. Ejaz H, Alsrhani A, Zafar A, Javed H, Junaid K, Abdalla AE, et al. COVID-19 and comorbidities: Deleterious impact on infected patients. J Infect Public Health [Internet]. Dec 2020 [cited 6 Dec 2022];13(12):1833-9. Available at: https://linkinghub.elsevier.com/retrieve/pii/S1876034120305943

35. Grasselli G, Greco M, Zanella A, Albano G, Antonelli M, Bellani G, et al. Risk Factors Associated With Mortality Among Patients With COVID-19 in Intensive Care Units in Lombardy, Italy. JAMA Intern Med [Internet]. 1 Oct 2020 [cited 6 Dec 2022];180(10):1345. Available from: https://jamanetwork.com/journals/jamainternalmedicine/fullarticle/2768601

36. Palaiodimos L, Kokkinidis DG, Li W, Karamanis D, Ognibene J, Arora S, et al. Severe obesity, increasing age and male sex are independently associated with worse in-hospital outcomes, and higher in-hospital mortality, in a cohort of patients with COVID-19 in the Bronx, New York. Metabolism [Internet]. July 2020 [cited 6 Dec 2022];108:154262. Available from: https://linkinghub.elsevier.com/retrieve/pii/S0026049520301268

37. Borobia A, Carcas A, Arnalich F, Álvarez-Sala R, Monserrat-Villatoro J, Quintana M, et al. A Cohort of Patients with COVID-19 in a Major Teaching Hospital in Europe. J Clin Med [Internet]. 4 June 2020 [cited 6 Dec 2022];9(6):1733. Available from: https://www.mdpi.com/2077-0383/9/6/1733

38. Pedersen HP, Hildebrandt T, Poulsen A, Uslu B, Knudsen HH, Roed J, et al. Initial experiences from patients with COVID-19 on ventilatory support in Denmark. 2020;4.

39. Metnitz PGH, Moreno RP, Fellinger T, Posch M, Zajic P. Evaluation and calibration of SAPS 3 in patients with COVID-19 admitted to intensive care units. Intensive Care Med [Internet]. August 2021 [cited 7 Dec 2022];47(8):910-2. Disponible sur: https://link.springer.com/10.1007/s00134-021-06436-9

40. Saida IB, Ennouri E, Nachi R, Meddeb K, Mahmoud J, Thabet N, et al. Very severe COVID-19 in the critically ill in Tunisia. Pan Afr Med J [Internet]. 2020 [cited 8 Dec 2022];35. Available from: https://www.panafrican-med-

journal.com/content/series/35/2/136/full

41. Lázaro APP, Albuquerque PLMM, Meneses GC, Zaranza M de S, Batista AB, Aragão NLP, et al. Critically ill COVID-19 patients in northeast Brazil: mortality predictors during the first and second waves including SAPS 3. Trans R Soc Trop Med Hyg [Internet]. 1 Nov 2022 [cited 7 Dec 2022];116(11):1054-62. Available at: https://academic.oup.com/trstmh/article/116/11/1054/6590401

42. Yang X, Yu Y, Xu J, Shu H, Xia J, Liu H, et al. Clinical course and outcomes of critically ill patients with SARS-CoV-2 pneumonia in Wuhan, China: a single-centered, retrospective, observational study. Lancet Respir Med [Internet]. May 2020 [cited 6 Dec 2022];8(5):475-81. Available at: https://linkinghub.elsevier.com/retrieve/pii/S2213260020300795

43. Pascarella G, Strumia A, Piliego C, Bruno F, Del Buono R, Costa F, et al. COVID-19 diagnosis and management: a comprehensive review. J Intern Med [Internet]. August 2020 [cited
7 Dec 2022];288(2):192-206. Available at: https://onlinelibrary.wiley.com/doi/10.1111/joim.13091

44. Raoof S, Nava S, Carpati C, Hill NS. High-Flow, Noninvasive Ventilation and Awake (Nonintubation) Proning in Patients With Coronavirus Disease 2019 With Respiratory Failure. Chest. Nov 2020;158(5):1992-2002.

45. Winck JC, Scala R. Non-invasive respiratory support paths in hospitalized patients with COVID-19: proposal of an algorithm. Pulmonology [Internet]. July 2021 [cited 8 Dec 2022];27(4):305-12. Available at: https://linkinghub.elsevier.com/retrieve/pii/S2531043720302658

46. Ferreyro BL, Angriman F, Munshi L, Del Sorbo L, Ferguson ND, Rochwerg B, et al. Association of Noninvasive Oxygenation Strategies With All-Cause Mortality in Adults With Acute Hypoxemic Respiratory Failure: A Systematic Review and Meta-analysis. JAMA. 7 Jul 2020;324(1):57-67.

47. Grieco DL, Menga LS, Cesarano M, Rosà T, Spadaro S, Bitondo MM, et al. Effect of Helmet Noninvasive Ventilation vs High-Flow Nasal Oxygen on Days Free of Respiratory Support in Patients With COVID-19 and Moderate to Severe Hypoxemic Respiratory Failure: The HENIVOT Randomized Clinical Trial. JAMA [Internet]. 4 May 2021 [cited 8 Dec 2022];325(17):1731. Available at: https://jamanetwork.com/journals/jama/fullarticle/2778088

48. Gupta S, Hayek SS, Wang W, Chan L, Mathews KS, Melamed ML, et al. Factors Associated With Death in Critically Ill Patients With Coronavirus Disease 2019 in the US. JAMA Intern Med [Internet]. Nov 1, 2020 [cited Dec 7, 2022];180(11):1436. Available from: https://jamanetwork.com/journals/jamainternalmedicine/fullarticle/2768602

49. AbdelGhaffar MM, Omran D, Elgebaly A, Bahbah EI, Afify S, AlSoda M, et al. Prediction of mortality in hospitalized Egyptian patients with Coronavirus disease-2019: A multicenter retrospective study. Mitra P, editor. PLOS ONE [Internet]. 11 Jan 2022 [cited 8 Dec2022];17(1):e0262348. Available from: https://dx.plos.org/10.1371/journal.pone.0262348

50. G G, E C, G F, M I, A Z, A C, et al. Mechanical ventilation parameters in critically ill COVID-19 patients: a scoping review. Crit Care Lond Engl [Internet]. 20 March 2021 [cited 1 May 2023];25(1). Available from: https://pubmed.ncbi.nlm.nih.gov/33743812/

51. COVID-ICU Group on behalf of the REVA Network and the COVID-ICU Investigators. Clinical characteristics and day-90 outcomes of 4244 critically ill adults with COVID-19: a prospective cohort study. Intensive Care Med. Jan 2021;47(1):60-73.

52. Baseline Characteristics and Outcomes of 1591 Patients Infected With SARS-CoV-2 Admitted to ICUs of the Lombardy Region, Italy - PubMed [Internet]. [cited 2 May 2023]. Available from: https://pubmed.ncbi.nlm.nih.gov/32250385/

53. Bardi T, Pintado V, Gomez-Rojo M, Escudero-Sanchez R, Azzam Lopez A, Diez-Remesal Y, et al. Nosocomial infections associated with COVID-19 in the intensive care unit: clinical characteristics and outcome. Eur J Clin Microbiol Infect Dis [Internet]. March 2021 [cited 10 Dec 2022];40(3):495-502. Available from: http://link.springer.com/10.1007/s10096-020-04142-w

54. Gabarre P, Dumas G, Zafrani L. Acute renal failure in COVID-19 patients in intensive care. :10.

55. Outcomes from intensive care in patients with COVID-19 a systematic review and meta analysis.pdf.

56. Grieco DL, Menga LS, Eleuteri D, Antonelli M. Patient self-inflicted lung injury: implications for acute hypoxemic respiratory failure and ARDS patients on non-invasive support. Minerva Anestesiol. Sep 2019;85(9):1014-23.

57. Meddeb K, Chelbi H, Boussarsar M. Fear, Preparedness and Covid-19. Tunis Med. May 2020;98(5):321-3.

58. Menga LS, Cese LD, Bongiovanni F, Lombardi G, Michi T, Luciani F, et al. High Failure Rate of Noninvasive Oxygenation Strategies in Critically Ill Subjects With Acute Hypoxemic Respiratory Failure Due to COVID-19. Respir Care. May 2021;66(5):705-14.

59. Weerakkody S, Arina P, Glenister J, Cottrell S, Boscaini-Gilroy G, Singer M, et al. Non-invasive respiratory support in the management of acute COVID-19 pneumonia: considerations for clinical practice and priorities for research. Lancet Respir Med. Feb 2022;10(2):199-213.

60. Wang JG, Liu B, Percha B, Pan S, Goel N, Mathews KS, et al. Cardiovascular Disease and Severe Hypoxemia Are Associated With Higher Rates of Noninvasive Respiratory Support Failure in Coronavirus Disease 2019 Pneumonia. Crit Care Explor [Internet]. 2021 [cited 4 May2023];e0355-e0355. Available at: https://www.ncbi.nlm.nih.gov/pmc/articles/PMC7909114

61. Grieco DL, Maggiore SM, Roca O, Spinelli E, Patel BK, Thille AW, et al. Non- invasive ventilatory support and high-flow nasal oxygen as first-line treatment of acute hypoxemic respiratory failure and ARDS. Intensive Care Med [Internet]. 2021 [cited 4 May 2023];47(8):851-66. Available at: https://www.ncbi.nlm.nih.gov/pmc/articles/PMC8261815/

62. Ben Dhia B, Essafi F, Ben Ismail K, Ben Slimene N, Bellardh H, Kaddour M, et al. Non-invasive ventilation in patients with COVID-19-related pneumonia: feasibility and clinical impact. Rev Mal Respir Actual [Internet]. 1 Dec 2021 [cited 5 May 2023];14(1):147-147. Available from: https://europepmc.org/articles/PMC8709596

63. Bertaina M, Nuñez-Gil IJ, Franchin L, Fernández Rozas I, Arroyo-Espliguero R, Viana-Llamas MC, et al. Non-invasive ventilation for SARS-CoV-2 acute respiratory failure: a subanalysis from the HOPE COVID-19 registry. Emerg Med J EMJ. May 2021;38(5):359-65.

64. Girault C. COVID-19 and acute respiratory failure: particularities of ventilatory management. Rev Mal Respir Actual [Internet]. 1 Dec 2022 [cited 3 Apr 2023];14(2, Supplement 2):2S483-91. Available at: https://www.sciencedirect.com/science/article/pii/S1877120322007856

65. Bahloul M, Kharrat S, Hafdhi M, Maalla A, Turki O, Chtara K, et al. Impact of prone position on outcomes of COVID-19 patients with spontaneous breathing. Acute Crit Care [Internet]. Aug 31, 2021 [cited Dec 8, 2022];36(3):208-14. Available from: http://accjournal.org/journal/view.php?doi=10.4266/acc.2021.00500

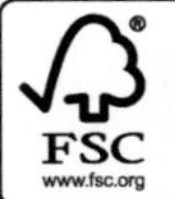

MIX
Papier aus verantwortungsvollen Quellen
Paper from responsible sources
FSC® C105338

Printed by Books on Demand GmbH, Norderstedt / Germany